Grapefruit Essential Oil

Benefits, Properties, Applications, Studies & Recipes

by Ann Sullivan

Published in USA by:

Ann Sullivan
217 N. Seacrest Blvd #9
Boynton Beach
FL 33425

© Copyright 2017

ISBN-13: ISBN-13: 978-1548104788
ISBN-10: 1548104787

Table of Contents

Introduction

What are essential oils, and how might they be used for therapeutic purposes?

Essential oils are ultra-potent oils, extracted from plants and flowers that have been utilized in medicine for centuries. Presently, they're most commonly used to supplement pharmaceutical medication, but they can also be an effective alternative to pharmaceuticals if you don't have access to them. Before you dismiss essential oils to support the body's natural defenses against injuries and illness, look at the historical evidence of the oils' therapeutic competence in practice. Your average age-old medical text will demonstrate that essential oils, herbs, and plenty of other natural ingredients have, for thousands of years, successfully enhanced immune function to meet and defeat any number of ailments and injuries. Though traditional medicine is considered "alternative" now, it was once the gold standard. And, frankly, perhaps it still should be, as these natural age-tested remedies can fortify the body's battlements against everything from simple maladies, like headaches, cuts and bruises, to serious diseases, like cancer.

Essential oils are deemed "essential," because the oils are composed of the "essence" of the plant. The difference between essential oils and other oils – like olive oil or vegetable oil, for instance – is that essential oils have high volatility and reduced fixation, which results in faster evaporation, enabling their popular use in aromatherapy.

Even at high temperatures, olive and vegetable oils don't evaporate.

Essential oils are especially necessary when it comes to a major natural or man-made disaster or some potential viral outbreak. In these types of dire situations, you may not have quick access (or any access at all) to your standard pharmaceutical supply; so, essential oils, along with other alternative medicines, will be your go-to wellness aids in the case of social collapse, viral outbreak or devastating natural disaster. When medical access is null and void, alternatives to our modern-day standard are the only chance we have to keep pathogens at bay.

You probably don't realize that you already use essential oils every day. They're in perfumes, shampoos, soaps, ointments...they're even used in furniture polish. Why are they found in so many aromatic products? Well, basically, because essential oils are super concentrated aromatic liquids, so their scent is remarkably strong. Let's put this into perspective: to steam tea, you use a few leaves of peppermint or juniper; to produce a single ounce of essential oil, five whole *pounds* of peppermint or juniper leaves are required. Some sources claim that to produce twelve pounds of essential oil would necessitate an acre of peppermint, juniper, or any other oil you're looking to produce en masse. Unlike vegetable oil, you don't often find concentrated therapeutic-grade essential oils sold in bulk; instead the oils are often sold in easily carried small, dark bottles, perfect for your GOOD bag (Get Out Of Dodge). Which is exactly what this book is aiming to help you do –

get out of dodge with your most vital of essential oils intact, a good supply of grapefruit essential oil.

Why grapefruit, you ask? Well, to get you quickly up to speed on this most essential of oils, below we've provided a condensed synopsis of grapefruit, after which we'll outline in greater detail the oil's history, properties, and common therapeutic uses, so that you – the consumer – might have a better understanding of the oil's benefits and applications. We've even provided supportive remedies for pure grapefruit, as well as blended recipes that incorporate the valuable oil. Chapter 3 will further detail past scientific research on grapefruit essential oil.

Now, let's get down to it.

Essential Oil 101: the Basics of Grapefruit

Summary: Grapefruit, or Citrus paradisi, has been traditionally used as a detoxifier. Grapefruit rids the body of toxins, including those from the lymphatic system. It can also help you lose weight, reduces water retention, and defends against cancer. The high amount of limonene in grapefruit essential oil means that it can be effective in protecting against stomach, pancreatic, skin, colon and liver cancers. In a study by Brigham Young University, grapefruit essential oil showed 80.5% inhibition against skin cancer cells, even in small concentrations. A study by Purdue University saw that the limonene aided the regression of breast cancer carcinomas by 80%.

Description: Grapefruit oil is commonly extracted

through cold pressed or expressed extraction. The rind or peel is most often used. The oil is yellow in color, thin in consistency, and has a somewhat strong sweet and tangy citrus scent.

Uses: Beyond those applications previously mentioned, additional uses for grapefruit essential oil include supporting the body's defenses against dull skin, acne, cellulitis, dyspepsia, toxin build-up, liver disorders, water retention, digestion, lymphatic decongestant, obesity, cleansing, hair, and Alzheimer's. When it comes to mood and emotion, grapefruit oil can combat anxiety and depression by uplifting the mind and body.

Properties: Antioxidant, antibacterial, antidepressant, antiseptic, disinfectant, diuretic, stimulant, and tonic properties.

Application: Dilute 1:1 with a carrier oil. You can apply topically, inhale directly, diffuse or use as a dietary supplement.

Safety Precautions: Grapefruit has been approved by the FDA for internal consumption and so can be used as a dietary supplement. Grapefruit is also photosensitive, so if used topically, avoid direct sunlight for up to 24 hours.

Fun facts: Grapefruit was originally known in Barbados as the "forbidden fruit." However, it was bred in Jamaica. In the 18th century, Captain Shaddock cultivated a hybrid mix of a fruit called pomelo and another called sweet orange. It was known there as the "shaddock" as a nod to its maker. Count Odette Philippe shipped the fruit to Florida in 1823.

Chapter 1 – Benefits of Grapefruit Essential Oil

Grapefruit essential oil offers several therapeutic benefits; but you may be wondering what these benefits are. In this chapter, we'll take a closer look at the history of grapefruit and its many uses.

Cultivation of Grapefruit

Citrus paradisi, otherwise known as grapefruit, is a semi-sweet and sour fruit, native to Barbados. It was borne as a hybrid of the pomelo and the sweet orange (C. maxima and C. sinensis, respectively). This species originates from evergreen trees that commonly grow up to 20 feet tall, and produce dark green leaves, white flowers and, of course, the yellowish orange fruit, with dimensions between 4 and 6 inches in diameter, on average. The acidic flesh varies in color, with pulps that also range from shades of red, pink and white between cultivators.

A History of Grapefruit

Original known as the "forbidden fruit," grapefruit has enjoyed a reputation as an especially delicious super fruit when it was first discovered. In fact, this hybrid fruit has an uncertain history. Some stories claim that grapefruit was a natural hybrid, bred on its own, while others claim Captain Shaddock came to Jamaica and planted some pomelo seeds, which bred the first grapefruit. In fact, up to the 19th century, grapefruits were also known as the "shaddocks." Its present-day name was derived from the fact that the fruit grows in grape-like clusters.

The fruit was considered of the most delicious taste and quality in Barbados and was documented in 1750 as "the forbidden fruit" for this very reason. It is still considered one of the "Seven Wonders of Barbados."

So how did grapefruit find its way around the world? In 1823, Count Odet Philippe brought the shaddocks to Florida, and more cross-hybrids were produced, including the tangelo. In the late 19th century, an American citrus industry entrepreneur and pioneer, named Kimball Chase Atwood, founded the Atwood Grapefruit Company and cultivated the largest grove of grapefruit the world over. This grove is responsible for breeding the pink grapefruit in 1906.

The Ruby Red grapefruit came along in 1929. Taking out the "inferior" white grapefruit in Texas, the Ruby now being a symbol and trademark of the state. Presently, Texas and Florida hold their own with grapefruit varieties, ranging from Ruby Red to Star Ruby to Oro Blanco. Their flavors also cover a wide range of acidity, from sweet to sour and tart. These differences are partially due to the grapefruit component called mercaptan, a terpene that contains sulfur and which is highly influential when it comes to the taste and the odor of the fruit.

Over the years, grapefruit has undergone a large amount of research, determining the nutritional content and the benefits of the fruit, as well as the mechanisms of its interactions with medication. Grapefruit is a rich source of vitamin C, fiber, and antioxidants, and it helps to lower cholesterol as well as to support the metabolism in burning fat, due to its low glycemic index. But the fruit has also been shown to interact adversely with several drugs, increasing the potency of drug compounds. This is due to the polyphenolic compounds found in grapefruit, particularly the flavanone, naringin, and the two furanocoumarins, dihydroxybergamottin and bergamottin, which inhibit CYP3A4, the drug-metabolizing enzyme found in the small intestine. By inhibiting this enzyme, the effects of certain drugs are more powerful, as they become more bioavailable. This may dissuade some from eating grapefruit or drinking grapefruit juice when on prescription medication; however, of the chemicals in question, naringin is not present in grapefruit essential oil, and the number of furanocoumarins found in the oil are not harmful, as they are significantly less than the volume present in grapefruit juice.

Despite these interactions with prescription drugs,

grapefruit has gained a reputation as one of the healthiest fruits. All the fruit's parts are used: the meat of the fruit for consumption, the peel for its essential oils, the pulp and seed by-product as cattle feed and for extract manufacturing. It is used not only in juices, but in jams in Haiti, and in desserts, such as toronja rellena in Costa Rica, a sweet that is stuffed with Dulce de Leche.

Nowadays, China is the largest producer of grapefruit, turning out around 3.8 million metric tons annually. The United States follows, producing about a third of China's scale, trailed by Mexico, Thailand, and South Africa.

Chemical Components

To generate the essential oil from grapefruit, the peel must be cold pressed. This results in the oil's key chemical components, which are primarily limonene, myrcene, linalool, terpinenol, neryl acetate, decyl acetate, geraniol, citronellal, sabinene, and alpha pinene.

Main Properties of Grapefruit Essential Oil

Along with the properties previously mentioned in the introduction, grapefruit oil possesses antioxidant, antibacterial, antidepressant, antiseptic, disinfectant, diuretic, stimulant, and tonic properties. With such a versatile range, grapefruit is well equipped to fight off any pathogen in the body's path.

Grapefruit, as mentioned, is composed of limonene, myrcene, linalool, terpinenol, neryl acetate, decyl acetate, geraniol, citronellal, sabinene, and alpha pinene. These components are what instill the enormously beneficial properties within grapefruit essential oil. We'll outline these properties below.

Antioxidant

Anything high in antioxidants – whether fruit, beans, or essential oils – is a powerful advocate for your body. Antioxidants both protect against free radicals and repair their damage. What are free radicals? Free radicals are destructive chemicals that invade your body, produced by substances both inside and out. Some free radicals (or oxidants) form through normal bodily reactions, like inflammation, metabolism and aerobic respiration. Other free radicals form outside the body, but enter it due to exposure. These include harmful pollutants, toxins, smoking, alcohol, X-rays, and UV rays, to name a few.

Although our bodies produce their own antioxidants, these often become damaged as we grow older; thus, introducing antioxidants into our bodies allows these nutrients and enzymes to assist in chemical reactions which destroy the oxidants or free radicals. Grapefruit essential oil is a moderate antioxidant, aiming to detox the body of free radicals that lead to disease.

Antibacterial

Grapefruit's antibacterial properties make it a powerful protectant against diseases produced by bacteria, such as oral, digestive and urinary tract bacterial infection. What's great is that, unlike some prescription drugs, grapefruit has no ill effects on bodily wellness or on the healthy natural flora that exists within the stomach and intestines.

Antidepressant

When it comes to psychological issues, the uplifting scent of grapefruit combats negative thoughts and, thereby, depression.

Antiseptic

The antiseptic and disinfectant properties of grapefruit essential oil can be reaped topically, applied directly to wounds, or even through burning; the smoke from the oil may help destroy airborne germs. Internal use will help keep the wounds from becoming infections, while external use will support the body's natural function in inhibiting tetanus.

Disinfectant

As a disinfectant, grapefruit can be added to household cleaners to disinfect your home. The oil eliminates contamination, which means your household will be healthier, overall, and will fall sick less often. Grapefruit can be used purely or blended with other oils to clean dishes, clothing, and practically any surface.

Diuretic

If you're looking to lose water weight and reduce blood pressure, grapefruit essential oil is your agent. The oil stimulates urination, promoting not only the loss of water weight, but the loss of fats, uric acid, sodium, and other body toxins.

Stimulant

Stimulants are often referred to as "uppers." This is because they produce mental or physical improvements or temporary enhancements of your bodily functions. For instance, you may grow more alert and awake or quicker on your feet after using a stimulant. Grapefruit essential oil can provide this temporary boost in mental and physical function, especially when it comes to the immune system.

Tonic

Grapefruit essential oil benefits each of the body's systems, whether nervous, digestive, respiratory or excretory, making it an unbeatable general tonic. The oil also supports the immune system by helping the body absorb nutrients.

Common Therapeutic Uses

Traditionally used to enhance the body's defenses against infections and diseases, grapefruit essential oil remains a significant immune system stimulant, protecting against several conditions, whether viral, fungal, or bacterial. Grapefruit supports overall wellness and organ function, while mentally uplifting and improving concentration. Let's take a closer look at the common uses for this oil.

Brain Stimulant

Grapefruit essential oil provides a refreshing and stimulating aroma that can relieve exhaustion and fatigue. It also produces mental focus and clarity, which is great when it comes to cognitive tasks, like studying or other brainwork.

Digestive Support

A healthy digestive tract means a healthy body, so maintaining good digestion can make a world of difference in overall wellness. Your digestive tract is between 25 and 30 feet long. If the length of it is not working properly, then there's a chance that food might get caught up along the tract and begin to rot within your body. Grapefruit effectively supports the digestive tracts' natural function by producing digestive juices and enzymes and inducing bile flow throughout the digestive organs. The oil also stimulates appetite, which makes it effective in combatting eating disorders, like anorexia.

Blood Pressure & Cardiovascular Wellness

Brimming with vitamins and minerals, especially vitamin C, grapefruit is also absent of sodium, which is a good thing when it comes to blood pressure. The oil's ability to reduce LDL cholesterol levels, along with its no-sodium/high-potassium balance positively impacts blood pressure and heart rate. The oil contains dietary fiber as well, which also helps to reduce bad cholesterol (LDL) and boost good cholesterol (HDL), resulting in better cardiovascular wellness. The oil's antioxidant properties and its ability to facilitate the dissolution of cholesterol that accumulates in arteries will also support cardiovascular issues, like heart disease or atherosclerosis.

Disinfectant & Cleanser

The fact that citrus oils are added to so many household cleaners doesn't come down to the fresh scent alone; being a disinfectant, grapefruit is the ultimate cleaning agent, because it eliminates contamination, deodorizes, bleaches, and destroys grease, and so can be used to clean dishes, clothing, and practically any surface.

Detoxifying Agent

Grapefruit essential oil is an effective detoxifying agent, for the lymphatic system. The oil's components eliminate oxidants that enter the body through such environmental inlets as the foods we eat, the products we use, the air we breathe, the water we wash with, and other like factors. Toxins can cause numerous physiological issues, including heart problems, lung or kidney diseases, or even cancer. What grapefruit does to eliminate free radicals is to draw the toxins out and transfer them into the urinary tract, where they can be safely removed from the body. Thus, through the oil's high antioxidant content and its ability to stimulate urination, grapefruit helps cleanse and detoxify the body's systems.

Immune System Booster

Grapefruit is a superb immune system support which boosts circulation and increases white blood cell count. The oil's chemical components deliver incredible antifungal properties, making it akin to an immune shield braced to fight off angry bacterial strains, like salmonella, E. coli and staph infections. With such strong armor, this immune stimulant will ensure that your body is better prepared to protect against deadly infections.

Skin Care

Grapefruit essential oil supports the body's defenses against acne, wrinkles, dryness, and other skin issues. The oil's properties invigorate dull skin, while cleansing and eliminating excess oil. Whether using grapefruit essential oil to defy skin aging or to reduce adolescent skin issues, like pimples and acne, the antiseptic, disinfectant, and antibacterial properties are superb for skin issues, no question.

Stress Disorders

Whether it be physical stress or mental stress, grapefruit essential oil's aroma, in conjunction with its therapeutic properties, enable its use in the support of stress disorders, like upset nerves, anxiety, melancholy, and depression. It can help soothe mental fatigue and refresh cognitive function. The oil induces restful sleep, stimulates concentration, and strengthens overall mental wellbeing.

Safety Precautions & Common Applications

Safety

Certain adverse effects may evolve when using pure essential oils. Some essential oils should not be used when pregnant, for example, as they may cause miscarriage. Allergic reactions, too, may occur, especially when applied topically. Always administer an allergy test before committing fully to topical application. When used with other medications, essential oils may react negatively. If you are on any current prescription medications or have a chronic illness, such as high blood pressure, epilepsy or liver disease, then researching the effects of essential oils against your own personal medical history will eliminate any potentially problematic issues.

Grapefruit has been approved by the FDA for internal consumption and so can be used as a dietary supplement. Citrus oils are photosensitive, so if applied topically, avoid direct sunlight for up to 24 hours. If you have sensitive skin, dilute heavily and test before extensive use. Otherwise, dilute 1:1 with a carrier oil. You can apply topically, diffuse or use as a dietary supplement.

Blends

Oftentimes, essential oils are manufactured as blends of several pure oils. For instance, the Protective Blend of certain brands is a mix of cinnamon, clove, rosemary, and eucalyptus. This blend can be used to boost the immune system to help support colds, viruses and flus. The downside to blends is that the more oils added to the mix, the higher the probability your patient may react negatively to the blend if he/she is prone to allergies. There is also the possibility of phototoxicity when working with blends, particularly if they include citrus oils. Be sure to read your labels before administering.

Regardless of these possible effects, essential oils are a viable option for supporting several conditions. Those looking to support or maintain their own personal wellness, or that of their families', should become educated on the uses of essential oils, their natural remedies and the methods of application. Only then can you begin building your kit of essential oils for survival.

Chapter 2 – Recipes for Grapefruit Essential Oil

In this chapter, we'll offer various recipes for grapefruit essential oil, both for pure grapefruit applications and blends. For pure applications, we've provided the appropriate dosage and method of administration to support specific ailments, from addiction to withdrawal. When it comes to blends, herbalists and aromatherapists often combine grapefruit essential oil with frankincense, bergamot, palmarosa, lavender, and geranium. We'll offer some fantastic blending options in the second half of this chapter.

Pure Applications

Addiction

To help combat addiction – whether drug, alcohol,

food, or otherwise –, dilute grapefruit essential oil in a 1:1 ratio with a carrier oil and apply topically, massaging over the solar plexus, the heart, the stomach, or the back of the neck. You can also place a drop of oil on the tip of the tongue and take internally, or administer aromatically, diffusing throughout the home or inhaling directly from the bottle.

Anorexia

Grapefruit can serve as an appetite stimulant by boosting the mood and promoting self-esteem, and so can support eating disorders, like anorexia. To administer, diffuse throughout the room.

Appetite Suppression

On the flipside, if grief, stress, illness, or depression causes you to overeat, diffusing grapefruit essential oil throughout the home can also curb cravings and suppress binge eating.

Bulimia

Again, grapefruit boosts self-esteem and mood, while balancing the appetite of those who suffer from depression or eating disorders. To administer, diffuse throughout the room.

Cardiovascular Support

To strengthen the body's defenses against heart issues, while enhancing cardiovascular wellness, dilute a drop of grapefruit essential oil in a 1:1 ratio with a carrier oil and massage into the area of the heart and the reflex points of the feet.

Cellulite

Diminish the appearance of cellulite by diluting 1-2 drops of grapefruit essential oil in a 1:1 ratio with a carrier oil and massaging the combo into the affected area in a kneading motion once a day.

Digestion

To aid digestion, place a drop in your drinking water several times daily. You can also apply topically by diluting grapefruit essential oil in a 1:1 ratio with a carrier oil and massaging it into the stomach.

Dry Throat

Eliminate dry throat by placing a drop of grapefruit essential oil into your drinking water. You can also try combining the oil with sea salts and warm water for a gargling solution.

Fatigue

Combat fatigue by diffusing grapefruit essential oil,

adding a few drops to your bathwater, or placing a drop of oil into your hands, rubbing your palms together, cupping them over your nose, and breathing deeply in and out for several minutes. You can also dilute in a 1:1 ratio with a carrier oil and apply in a full body massage or over your chest. The oil will increase blood circulation, which will boost energy and brain function.

Edema

To relieve leg or feet swelling or edema due to hot/humid weather, combine 1-2 drops of grapefruit essential oil in a 1:1 ratio with a carrier oil and massage into the affected area, toward the heart, up to three times daily. Apply topically for three days, once in the morning, once midday, and once in the evening to the outside of the leg, from the knee up to above the waist.

Gallbladder Stones

Support the body's natural defenses against gallbladder stone issues by diluting 1 to 2 drops of grapefruit essential oil in a 1:1 ratio with a carrier oil, then apply topically, massaging it over the affected area and into the reflex points of the feet, three times daily.

Hangovers

Need a quick hangover fix? Dilute grapefruit essential oil in a 1:1 ratio with a carrier oil and massage it into the abdomen, chest, and the reflex points on your hands and feet. You can also diffuse, inhale directly, add a drop to drinking water, or place a few drops in your bathwater.

Jet Lag

Combat jet lag by diluting grapefruit essential oil in a 1:1 ratio with a carrier oil, then apply topically in a full-body massage. You can also inhale directly or diffuse throughout the room to refresh your senses after a long journey.

Kidney Support

Support the body's natural defenses against kidney issues by diluting grapefruit essential oil in a 1:1 ratio with a carrier oil and apply topically, massaging it over the affected area, three times daily. You can also add a drop or two to your drinking water and take internally.

Liver Support

Support liver function by diluting grapefruit essential oil in a 1:1 ratio with a carrier oil; then apply topically, massaging over the affected area and into the reflex points of the feet. You can also place a drop in your drinking water and take internally daily.

Lymphatic System Cleanse

To cleanse the lymphatic system, grapefruit essential oil can be applied topically to induce sweating. Simply add a drop to your lotion and massage into your body, starting at your extremities and moving toward the heart.

Stress

Combat stress by steaming two drops of grapefruit essential oil in a pan of water, remove the steaming pan from the stove, pour into a bowl, place a towel over your head and inhale. If you don't feel it's done its job the first time, you can reheat that same water and use it once more without adding more oil. You can also diffuse, add several drops to your bathwater, place a drop onto your shirt collar for portable stress relief, or apply topically, diluting in a 1:1 ratio with a carrier oil and massaging over the heart and solar plexus.

Migraines

Migraines can be relieved with grapefruit essential oil. Diffuse throughout the room or, for a more direct application, dilute the oil in a 1:1 ratio with a carrier oil and apply topically over the area of pain, into the temples and the base of the neck. Avoid the eyes.

Miscarriage (After)

Following a miscarriage, grapefruit can support both

physical and emotional support. Dilute in a 1:1 ratio with a carrier oil and use in a full-body massage and into the reflex points of the feet.

Obesity

Although grapefruit essential oil can be used as an appetite stimulant, it can also be used to help lose weight, as it promotes urination and detoxification. Add a few drops to your drinking water throughout the day and, for added support, diffuse throughout the home.

Overeating

Similarly, keep from overeating by diffusing grapefruit essential oil throughout the home. You can also put a drop on your shirt collar or place a drop in your palms, rub your hands together, and run them through your hair.

PMS

Relieve PMS symptoms by diffusing throughout your cycle. You can also dilute grapefruit essential oil in a 1:1 ratio with a carrier oil and massage it into the solar plexus, the lower abdomen, and the reflex points of the feet on a regular basis throughout the month.

Sugar Cravings

Keep those sugar cravings at bay by diffusing grapefruit essential oil throughout the home. You can also put a drop on your shirt collar, inhale directly, add a few drops to your drinking water, or place a drop in your palms, rub your hands together, and run them through your hair.

Withdrawal

Combat issues of withdrawal by diluting grapefruit essential oil in a 1:1 ratio with a carrier oil and apply topically, massaging it over the throat. For added support, you can also diffuse the oil throughout the home.

Blends

Alert Stimulant

Ingredients

- 4 drops Juniper Berry Essential Oil
- 5 drops Grapefruit Essential Oil
- 6 drop Ginger Essential Oil
- 15 mL Carrier Oil

Directions

To promote alertness, clarity, and energy, place all ingredients into a bowl, blending well. Apply topically in a full-body massage.

Anti-Anxiety Bath

Ingredients

- 2 drops Basil Essential Oil
- 2 drops Grapefruit Essential Oil
- 2 drops Geranium Essential Oil
- 3 drops Lavender Essential Oil
- 3 drops Ylang Ylang Essential Oil

Directions

To wind down, de-stress, and combat anxiety, add all ingredients to your bathwater and stir to disperse. Then inhale deeply while you soak for 20 minutes, but avoid getting water in your eyes, as it may sting.

Cirrhosis of the Liver

Ingredients

- 2 drops Grapefruit Essential Oil
- 2 drops Clove Essential Oil
- 1 drop Geranium Essential Oil
- 1 drop Rosemary Essential Oil
- 1 tsp Carrier Oil

Directions

To support the liver and combat cirrhosis, combine all ingredients and apply topically over the region of the liver twice daily.

Citrus Oil Detoxifier

Ingredients

- 1 drop Tangerine Essential Oil
- 1 drops Lemon Essential Oil
- 1 drop Grapefruit Essential Oil
- 24 ounces Water (separated)

Directions

Drinking plenty of water throughout the day is not only a good way to stay hydrated and healthy, but it also flushes out toxins, which interfere with hormonal balance. Citrus oils are particularly beneficial to cleansing the body (particularly the lymphatic system) of these toxins. Add a single drop of one of the oils to each 8 ounces of drinking water throughout the day to reduce toxins, aid hormone balance, and increase libido.

De-stress Bath

Ingredients

- 2 drops Rosemary Essential Oil
- 3 drops Black Pepper Essential Oil
- 5 drops Grapefruit Essential Oil
- 1 Tbsp. Grapeseed Oil

Directions

To wind down, de-stress, and combat anxiety, add all ingredients to your bathwater and stir to disperse. Then inhale deeply while you soak for 20 minutes, but avoid getting water in your eyes, as it may sting.

Detoxifying Blend I

Ingredients

- 2 drops Juniper Berry Essential Oil
- 2 drops Lavender Essential Oil
- 2 drops Grapefruit Essential Oil
- 2 drops Basil Essential Oil
- 2 drops Cypress Essential Oil
- 30 mL Carrier Oil

Directions

To flush out toxins and boost circulation, combine all ingredients, blending well, and massage into the reflex points in the feet.

Detoxifying Blend II

Ingredients

- 6 drops Juniper Berry Essential Oil
- 8 drops Lemon Essential Oil
- 8 drops Grapefruit Essential Oil
- 3.5 ounces Carrier Oil

Directions

Detoxify the body's systems by combining all ingredients in a small bowl or container and blend well. Apply topically, massaging into the specific reflex points of your feet, depending upon the organ you wish to detoxify, or in a full-body massage.

Fungal Infections

Ingredients

- 3 drops Grapefruit Essential Oil
- 2 drops Cinnamon Essential Oil
- 1 drop Basil Essential Oil
- 1 drop Patchouli Essential Oil
- ½ ounce Carrier Oil

Directions

To eliminate fungal infections, combine all ingredients and apply topically to affected area.

Gluten Intolerance

Ingredients

- 1 drop Cinnamon Bark Essential Oil
- 2 drops Grapefruit Essential Oil
- 2 drops Ginger Essential Oil
- 2 drops Lemon Essential Oil

Instructions

To help strengthen the body's natural defenses against gluten intolerance, place all ingredients into a "00" capsule, and ingest 1 capsule a day.

Liver Cleanse

Ingredients

- 4 drops Rosemary Essential Oil
- 4 drops Lemongrass Essential Oil
- 4 drops Grapefruit Essential Oil

Directions

To cleanse the liver, place all ingredients into a "00" capsule, and ingest 1 capsule a day.

Lymphatic Cleanse

Ingredients

- 3 drops Cypress Essential Oil
- 2 drops Grapefruit Essential Oil
- 1 drop Orange Essential Oil
- 1 Tbsp. Carrier Oil

Directions

To cleanse the lymphatic system, combine all ingredients in a small bowl and blend well. Apply topically, massaging over the lymph area and into the reflex points of the feet.

Stress-Reducing Massage Oil

Ingredients

- 1 Tbsp. Carrier Oil
- 1 drop Lavender Essential Oil
- 3 drops Cinnamon Bark Essential Oil
- 3 drops Grapefruit Essential Oil
- 4 drops Fennel Essential Oil
- 4 drops Roman Chamomile Essential Oil
- 5 drops Melissa Essential Oil

Directions

In a small bowl or jar, combine oils, mixing until evenly distributed. Massage the oil into the shoulders, back and neck. Recommended for two-time use before a stressful event, 6 hours apart to help relieve anxiety.

Stress Relief

Ingredients

- 25 drops Wild Orange Essential Oil
- 20 drops Grapefruit Essential Oil
- 15 drops Frankincense Essential Oil
- 15 drops Bergamot Essential Oil
- 10 drops Clary Sage Essential Oil
- 10 drops Lemon Essential Oil

Directions

To help focus concentration, combine ingredients in a bottle. Diffuse 6-7 drops as needed throughout the home or office.

Weight loss

Ingredients

- 2 drop Lemons Essential Oil
- 2 drops Grapefruit Essential Oil
- 2 drops Peppermint Essential Oil

Instructions

To promote weight loss, place all ingredients into a "00" capsule, and ingest 1 capsule twice a day.

Chapter 3 – Grapefruit Essential Oil Studies

Many studies have been done on essential oils to uncover and prove their therapeutic qualities. In the case of the great number of grapefruit studies, many of the properties attributed to the essential oil (noted in this book and elsewhere) are quite often validated through the research from accredited universities and published by reputable scientific journals. In this chapter, we'll discuss a small portion of these studies. It's important to note that research on essential oils is constantly evolving. Keep up with any recent research, as it may turn up even further valuable uses for these miracle oils.

Study 1 – Acne & Cancer

In this study published by *Molecules*, grapefruit essential oil's effects on acne and cancer cells were examined, with the following results: "Ten essential oils, (including grapefruit (Citrus paradisi Macf., Rutaceae)) were tested for their antibacterial activities towards Propionibacterium acnes and in vitro toxicology against three human cancer cell lines...The cytotoxicity of 10 essential oils on human prostate carcinoma cell (PC-3) was significantly stronger than on human lung carcinoma (A549) and human breast cancer (MCF-7) cell lines."

This study tested grapefruit essential oil, along with several other essential oils, against Propionibacterium acnes, the Gram-positive bacterium responsible for acne and other skin conditions. The study also evaluated the essential oil's effects on lung cancer, breast cancer, and prostate cancer. The antibacterial properties of grapefruit essential oil were midrange amongst the oils, killing 100% of P. acnes after thirty minutes in a .25% concentration. As for the cancer cell lines, grapefruit, and particularly the oil's aldehyde compounds, showed cytotoxicity against the HL-60 cells cancer cells, otherwise known as leukemia cells. This study indicates that grapefruit can be effectively utilized in supporting the body's natural defenses against acne and leukemia.

Reference

http://www.ncbi.nlm.nih.gov/pubmed/20657472]

http://www.mdpi.com/1420-3049/15/5/3200]

Study 2 – Antibacterial Properties

In this study published by *Evidence-Based Complementary and Alternative Medicine*, the antibacterial effects of grapefruit essential oil were examined, with the following results: "Hospital-acquired infections and antibiotic-resistant bacteria continue to be major wellness concerns worldwide. Particularly problematic is methicillin-resistant Staphylococcus aureus (MRSA) and its ability to cause severe soft tissue, bone or implant infections…Several common and hospital-acquired bacterial and yeast isolates (6 Staphylococcus strains including MRSA, 4 Streptococcus strains and 3 Candida strains including Candida krusei) were tested for their susceptibility for…Grapefruit…Remarkably, almost all tested oils demonstrated efficacy against hospital-acquired isolates and reference strains, whereas Olive and Paraffin oil from the control group produced no inhibition. As proven in vitro, essential oils represent a cheap and effective antiseptic topical treatment option even for antibiotic-resistant strains as MRSA and antimycotic-resistant Candida species."

S. aureus is Gram-positive bacterium. Methicillin-resistant Staphylococcus aureus (MRSA) is any strain of S. aureus that's naturally developed a resistance to antibiotics, including penicillin. This hospital-acquired infection is now limitedly endemic. Being resistant to standard medications, these strains – although not more virulent than other S. aureus strains – may result in infections that are tough to treat. Hospitals, nursing homes, and prisons largely house

MRSA, and patients with weak immune systems and open wounds are most at risk.

Streptococcus strains are Gram-positive bacteria as well. Depending on the strain, this bacteria can potentially result in fatal infections.

The study also tested the oils against Candida strains, which are fungi or yeast. Candida krusei is a yeast primarily used in chocolate production, though it may have fungal pathogen like effects in immunocompromised individuals.

The study found that grapefruit essential oil, along with all other oils tested, had an inhibitory effect on the MRSA strain, the other Staphylococcus and Streptococcus strains, and the Candida strains, without any cytotoxic effect on skin cells. These results indicate that grapefruit essential oil could potentially be used as an antibacterial and antifungal agent against the strains tested.

Reference
http://www.ncbi.nlm.nih.gov/pubmed/19473851]

Study 3 – Insecticidal Properties

In this study available on PubMed, the insecticidal activity of grapefruit essential oil was examined, with the following results: "Laboratory bioassay of the essential oil extracted from the grapefruit (Citrus paradisi) peel by steam distillation was carried out against the developmental stages of the yellow fever vector Aedes aegypti to evaluate its toxicity, and ovicidal and larvicidal potency...The results indicated that the peel oil could be a potent persistent larvicide."

Prevalent primarily in the tropics, yellow fever – otherwise known as dengue fever – affects between 50 and 528 million people annually and is endemic in over 110 countries. The infection is transmitted via mosquitoes which carry the dengue virus. The resulting symptoms of the viral disease include joint and muscle pain, fever, and skin rash which is akin to the measles. The disease can sometimes escalate into dengue hemorrhagic fever or dengue shock syndrome, each far more fatal than common dengue fever. There is no commercial vaccine for dengue fever, therefore eliminating the mosquitoes' habitats and reducing exposure to bites is the primary preventative measure. Treatment of dengue fever, as well, is supported primarily through rehydration with no pharmaceutical medication yet developed to target the virus directly (although medications are in development).

Grapefruit essential oil shows promise in the preventative department. The oil demonstrated superior inhibitory properties against the larvae of Ae. aegypti, the mosquito species that commonly carries the virus. At 400ppm, egg hatching was completely inhibited, making grapefruit essential oil an effective potential mosquito control in areas where dengue fever is endemic.

Reference

http://www.ncbi.nlm.nih.gov/pubmed/24450234]

Study 4 – Post-Menopausal Wellness

In this study published by *BMC Complementary & Alternative Medicine*, the effects of grapefruit essential oil on the abdominal fat and body image of post-menopausal women were examined, with the following results: "The purpose of this study was to verify the effect of aromatherapy massage on abdominal fat and body image in post-menopausal women…The results suggest that Aromatherapy massage could be utilized as an effective intervention to reduce abdominal subcutaneous fat, waist circumference, and to improve body image in post-menopausal women."

The study involved two groups of women, a control and an experimental group. Each received a body massage treatment for one hour, once a week for six weeks. The women in the control group were massaged with grapeseed oil, while those in the experimental group received a cypress-grapefruit blend. The study's objective was to evaluate the effect of aromatherapy massage on abdominal fat and body image in the subjects.

Data was collected pre- and post-test from both groups, including physical measurements and psychological wellness tests, and the results demonstrated that the waist circumference and abdominal subcutaneous fat were reduced more in the experimental group than in the control group. Body image had also improved more in the experimental group. These results indicate that grapefruit essential oil can be used in aromatherapy massage to improve body image and decrease waist circumference and abdominal subcutaneous fat in post-menopausal women.

Reference
http://www.ncbi.nlm.nih.gov/pubmed/17615482]

Study 5 – Antioxidant Properties

In this study published by *Natural Product Research*, the antioxidant activity of grapefruit essential oil was examined, with the following results: "The antioxidant activities and the determined major components of six popular and commercially available herb essential oils, including lavender (Lavendular angustifolia), peppermint (Mentha piperita), rosemary (Rosmarius officinalis), lemon (Citrus limon), grapefruit (Citrus paradise), and frankincense (Boswellia carteri), were compared…The highest DPPH radical-scavenging activity was obtained by the lavender essential oil and limonene, with RC50 values of 2.1 +/- 0.23% and 2.1 +/- 0.04%, respectively."

As mentioned in the study abstract, this was a comparative study of the antioxidant activities of several oils and their main components. Antioxidants protect against free radicals and repair their damage. Although our bodies produce their own antioxidants, these often become damaged as we age, so introducing antioxidants into our bodies allows these nutrients and enzymes to assist in chemical reactions which destroy the oxidants or free radicals. Grapefruit's main component is limonene, which composes 94.2% of the oil's content. Limonene was shown to have significant antioxidant properties, amongst the highest of all oils tested, indicating grapefruit essential oil's efficacy as an antioxidant agent.

Study 6 – Leukemia

In this study published by *In Vivo*, the anticancer activity of grapefruit essential oil was examined, with the following results: "Limonene is a primary component of citrus essential oils (EOs) and has been reported to induce apoptosis on tumor cells. Little is known about induction of apoptosis by citrus EOs. In this study, we examined induction of apoptosis by…Citrus paradisi (grapefruit)…These EOs induced apoptosis in HL-60 cells and the apoptosis activities were related to the limonene content of the EOs."

This study evaluated the viability of grapefruit essential oil in inhibiting leukemia cells. Leukemia is a type of cancer caused by invariable factors, including both environmental and inherited. The cancer is created by the accumulation of many abnormal white blood cells, starting in the bone marrow. These underdeveloped white blood cells cause symptoms of increased fatigue, bruising, bleeding, and risk of infection. The cancer is the most common type for children, though about 90% of the cases occur in adults, with 265,000 global deaths in 2012, alone.

In the study, citrus essential oils were tested on leukemia cancer cells, due to their limonene content, which is said to induce apoptosis in these cells. In multicellular organisms, apoptosis is the process of programmed cell death. In the case of cancer, an insufficient amount of apoptosis results in an unmanageable growth of cancer cells, thus the cell death induced by the citrus essential oils tested may be applicable to controlling the cancer's growth. Grapefruit was found to have additional apoptotic components over and above limonene. Decanal, octanal and citral demonstrated strong apoptotic activity, as well, which indicates that the aldehyde compounds may also be responsible for grapefruit's powerful apoptotic inhibition of HL-60 cells. The results suggest that grapefruit essential oil may potentially be used to support the body's defenses against leukemia cancer growth.

Reference http://www.ncbi.nlm.nih.gov/pubmed/14758720]

Chapter 4 – The Ins & Outs of Essential Oils

Where do essential oils come from?

Plants and plant species naturally produce essential oils for various reasons, one being to draw pollinator insects to them, another being to repel invading organisms (bacteria, animals). Many chemical compounds compose each plant's essential oil, and the combination of these compounds are specific to each oil, which then instills in the oil its own unique properties. Essential oils can be harnessed from all sorts of plant components, including flowers, leaves, bark, fruit, roots, and resin. For instance, cinnamon oil is harnessed from bark, lemon oil from the peel, and lavender oil from lavender flowers. Certain plants can produce a few chemical variants of the same essential oil, which are acquired from different parts of the plant. Some of these parts produce a large amount of oil, while others produce just a smidgen. The oil's quality and potency depends upon several factors, including the subspecies of the plant, its soil conditions, the time of year and even the time of day you harvest it.

How are essential oils extracted?

Essential oils can be extracted from plants through various methods, including pressing, distillation, solvent and maceration. Let's take a brief look at each:

Pressing Method

Commonly used with citrus fruit, the pressing method extracts the oil through a technique which involves pushing the fruit peels through a press. Oily fruits and plants are best suited for this technique. Orange oil, for example, is extracted from orange skins through the pressing method.

Distillation Method

This technique harkens back to the days of old-timey moonshiners, as the same sort of method used to create strong liquor can be used to extract essential oils. Using a still, boiled water and plant materials will create steam which is then cooled by coils and condensed into a combination of water and oil. This combination doesn't mix, so the oil can then be extracted from it.

Solvent Method

Through a multi-step process, certain plant and flower oils can be extracted using alcohol and other solvents, which extort the essential oil from the plant materials.

Maceration Method

When a "carrier" or fixed oil or lard is mixed with the plant material and set out in the sun, over a period, the carrier oil is infused with the plant's essence. Heat sources, other than the sun, are often used to speed the process. Throughout the process, more plant material is added to produce a more potent oil.

How do you use essential oils?

Although some studies about the effectiveness of essential oils are conducted by small companies or even individuals, several them are conducted by the food and cosmetic industries. In general, the pharmaceutical industry shows next to no interest in herbal medicine, primarily because there are few options to patent such products. Being as such, the product's lack of profitability results in a lack of research funding. Regardless, the historical uses of essential oils tell us what we need to know: these oils have been effectively administered for centuries. The therapeutic qualifications of essential oils can be plotted in the survival of humans across cultures and generations.

Another reason that studies on essential oils have not resulted in much conclusive evidence as to their overall effectiveness is because definitive results are sometimes difficult to prove, as the quality of each batch of oil can vary for several reasons. One is that essential oils are impossible to standardize. As mentioned above, even the slightest variance in soil conditions and the time of harvesting – as well as innumerable other factors – will produce a different product quality and potency. In addition, essential oils are often obtained from various species of the same plant; Eucalyptus radiata and Eucalyptus globulus can both be used in the making of therapeutic-grade eucalyptus oil and, as a result, they may have slightly different properties and degrees of strength or effectiveness.

Just as there are several methods by which to extract essential oils, there are many methods to administer them therapeutically. The variety of chemical compounds in each essential oil means that their benefits and applications also vary across the board. Below are a few of these methods.

Topical Administration

Direct application of many essential oils works like a sponge, as skin sops up chemicals and other things (like sunlight, for instance). Topical application is best when you want to clear up an ailment on the skin's surface or in the underlying muscle tissue. When applying topically, you may either massage the oil into the skin or simply dab on the skin for therapeutic results. You might combine the essential oil with a carrier oil for topical use to dilute its potency. This is safer, as the oil is so concentrated. You may support your body's defenses against rash or muscle pain in this manner, but you should always test your patient for allergens before applying. Adverse effects are produced by natural chemicals as much as synthetic ones; poison ivy, for example.

To test for allergens, place a drop or two on your patient's inner forearm. If a rash develops within 12 to 24 hours, then the patient is allergic. In addition, phototoxicity – sun exposure resulting in an exacerbated burn – may be an issue when citrus oils are applied topically. So, one must proceed with caution when applying essential oils using this method.

Inhalation Therapy

Commonly known as "aromatherapy", this essential oil application is effective for inner ailments, like sore throat or cold. In a steaming bowl of distilled or sterilized water, add a few drops of essential oil and, with a towel over your head, bend over the bowl and inhale. The towel captures the vapors, making the technique even more effective. Essential oils can also be placed in a diffuser or potpourri throughout a room to produce somewhat diluted therapeutic effects.

Ingestion

When using this method, proceed with caution. Direct ingestion of essential oils must be monitored and applied in small doses that are diluted in a tablespoon or more of any carrier oil – olive oil, for example. If you are unsure of dosage amounts, make a tea with the relevant herb instead. Although the effects of this diluted use may be weaker, this application is a better alternative than an overdose of essential oils.

What are the general benefits of using essential oils?

Replacement for Prescription Drugs

One practical benefit for using essential oils is, of course, their substitutive nature. Many believe that they can replace Rx drugs, which is the ultimate reason to educate yourself on their application and to begin stockpiling your essential oil supply. Although it is our opinion that 100% pure essential oils that carry no harmful side effects are better to support the body and its functions, we recommend that you consult your physician before replacing your prescription or over-the-counter medications.

One of the potential threats of economic or social collapse is the lack of resources, and primarily the inability to procure prescription drugs. Being as such, finding suitable alternatives should be a priority when prepping for the worst.

Their portability is also a major bonus when it comes to survival prepping. The fact that these ultra-concentrated oils take up little-to-no space makes toting them to your shelter all the simpler should the need arise. And, because essential oils are highly concentrated, the application used in most procedures requires only a drop or two of oil, which means that tiny bottle will be long-lasting (example 15mL bottle contains approx. 250 drops).

Cheap, but Effective Alternative

Though money may be the last thing on your mind when it comes to prepping for a survival situation (money may even be obsolete in the event of social collapse), it is worth noting that the expense of essential oils pales in comparison to prescription drugs. In fact, whether you are forced to survive on essential oils due to a lack of prescription reserves, in some cases, you might consider substituting your prescriptions for these inexpensive alternatives regardless. Essential oils are a cheap, but equally effective alternative to prescription medicine.

No Expiration Date

Another benefit of essential oils is that they do not expire, neither do they have "proper storage" requirements. Several medicines and therapeutic products must be replaced every couple years, so this sets essential oils ahead of the pack when it comes to shelf life.

Versatility

Essential oils also offer great versatility. Apart from providing wellness benefits, essential oils can be repurposed for household and hygienic applications. For instance, if you're looking for something that might serve your dental hygiene needs in a time of crisis, thieves oil is your go-to essential oil. If you want to maintain your skin's wellness, frankincense and lavender will do the trick; the latter also serves as sunscreen, so you can prevent sun damage as well.

When it comes to the house or shelter, you can use essential oils to deodorize, which will come in handy in a disaster scenario where things might start to smell fishy due to lack of proper utilities and care. For example, after the 2011 tsunami and the subsequent nuclear reactor meltdown in Japan, a nurse named Risa Nakahira used essential oils to deodorize and sanitize putrid public bathrooms in overpopulated evacuation facilities. As relief workers searched for survivors, often wading through debris and decay, Nakahira also deodorized their boots and masks using essential oils. The possibilities of these natural oils are endless.

They are also versatile when it comes to the range of patients they're capable of supporting. The wellness of everyone from your great grandfather to your infant baby can be fortified with the aid of essential oils in the appropriate dosage. They even come in handy when supporting livestock or pets. From teething infants to dementia in the elderly, from teenagers with acne to dogs with urinary tract infections, essential oils can serve any patient with nearly any ailment.

Conclusion

Now that you know all about what grapefruit essential oil can do for you – where it originates, how it's extracted, its benefits and properties, and the different methods of administration – you can use it confidently to support the body's defenses against wellness issues and start to assemble a kit of essential oils for survival.

The various benefits of essential oils and their properties are countless. To build your own kit, first focus on acquiring the essential oils which may bear more relevance to your wellness issues or the potential wellness threats within your environment. When it comes to stress disorders, for instance, grapefruit essential oil will be one of your more crucial oils, due to its uplifting and stimulating properties.

Used as a supplement or as your go-to for detoxification, skin care, or immune system support, the application of grapefruit essential oil in medicine has survived for centuries and will survive centuries more. When it comes down to it, you don't need to rely on pharmaceuticals; essential oils, herbs, and plenty of other natural ingredients can be used to help support any number of wellness issues, whether ailment or injury.

Essential oils are essential to your survival in the case of viral outbreak, social collapse or natural disaster because, when the SHTF, your access to pharmaceuticals will likely either be limited or eliminated altogether. Alternatives to our modern-day standard will equate survival when no other option exists. And when it comes to a life-or-death situation, you can't let your wellness decline, no matter the state of the world.

DISCLAIMER AND/OR LEGAL NOTICES: Every effort has been made to accurately represent this book and it's potential. Results vary with every individual, and your results may or may not be different from those depicted. No promises, guarantees or warranties, whether stated or implied, have been made that you will produce any specific result from this book. Your efforts are individual and unique, and may vary from those shown. Your success depends on your efforts, background and motivation.

The material in this publication is provided for educational and informational purposes only and is not intended as medical advice. The information contained in this book should not be used to diagnose or treat any illness, metabolic disorder, disease or health problem. Always consult your physician or healthcare provider before beginning any nutrition or exercise program. Use of the programs, advice, and information contained in this book is at the sole choice and risk of the reader.